KETO DIET QUICK

THE KETO DIET BOOK WITH QUICK AND HEALTHY RECIPES INCL. 3 WEEKS WEIGHT LOSS AND MEAL PLAN

KATE L. TAYLOR

D1556061

ISBN- 9798617934184

TABLE OF CONTENTS

INTRODUCTION

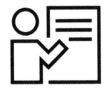

This precious book is going to change you forever. It is for those people who want to lose weight and lead a healthy lifestyle. The keto diet is a wonderful opportunity to turn you into a better healthier self.

This book, I hope, will be exciting, beautiful and smart for you to read. You are sure to make new discoveries each and every day.

This book presents a set of recommendations and tips on how to eat healthily and be slim.

Enjoy reading!

The author

THE KETO DIET: ALL ABOUT IT

A keto diet is a low-carbohydrate diet, which helps to lose weight effectively by producing ketones in the liver which are used as energy. Ketones are special chemicals which are produced in the human liver. They appear when there is not enough insulin in the body to turn sugar or glucose into energy. In this case, the body uses fat and turns it into ketones. Then it sends them up into blood.

This diet is called differently in various books and publications but the most common names for it are as follows: the Keto diet, low-carb diet, low-carb high-fat diet and others.

To understand the principle on which this diet is based, let's look on the mechanisms of energy generation in our body. The first and foremost energy source for our organism is surely glucose. When something high in carbohydrates is consumed, the human body turns it into glucose, which then increases the levels of sugar in blood. To stabilise the amount of glucose in the human body, pancreas produces the substance called insulin.

Glucose is the simplest molecule which generates energy in the human body. Insulin processes this molecule by moving it in the body. The glucose is the main energy source, so fats are stored in the body since they are not necessary.

When a person has a high carbohydrate diet, the body uses glucose as the major energy source. By reducing carbohydrates taken in, the body gets into ketosis. What is "ketosis"?

Ketosis is a usual state of a human's body, which starts when there is too little glucose in food. At this time, the body starts to produce ketones to provide human beings with a sufficient energy level and nutrition for brain cells.

The main aim of the keto diet is to turn the human's body into the state of "ketosis". It is vital to stress that the process is triggered by a very low amount of carbohydrates in meals.

There are a lot of pros for our health when we have the necessary number of ketones and low sugar level in our bloodstream: firstly, the state of health will greatly improve; secondly, there will be a decrease in fat stored in the human body; thirdly, the human being will be more concentrated and the last but not the least factor is that a person will be full of energy and vitality, which is really a very positive side of the keto diet.

A keto diet presupposes that you take in a lot of fat, a moderate protein amount and a very low carbohydrate amount.

Your diet should include about 70% of fat, 25% of protein and only 5% of carbohydrates.

HOW TO LOSE WEIGHT BEING ON THE KETO DIET

Keto diet will surely help you to lose weight and make positive changes in your lifestyle.

After a couple of weeks on the keto diet, our body will be good at burning fat and using ketones for energy instead of carbohydrates. The keto diet also decreases insulin levels. So we can say that this diet is a healthy option for those eager to lose weight and be healthy.

Meat, cheese, oils, fish, butter, nuts, avocadoes, and seeds are examples of foods which are recommended when on the diet.

Almost all carbohydrate sources are to be thrown away from your diet, including rice, grains, beans, potatoes, milk, cereals, and fruits.

You should remember – this diet doesn't restrict calorie intake – in this case the keto diet helps you to lose weight by putting your body into ketosis. As we mentioned before, when you consume a small amount of carbohydrates, your body produces ketones for energy.

When on the keto diet, human body starts burning fat as an energy source and then you will begin to lose weight. And most importantly, the keto diet can fight the belly fat which many people struggle to eliminate.

Belly fat, or as it is also called the visceral fat, comes from a mix of genes and a diet high in carbohydrates and sugar. Visceral fat can easily become inflamed, making it extremely stubborn to lose and dangerous to blood vessels.

It is advisable to combine keto diet with high-intensity interval training exercises.

Being on the diet, you should take into account the fact that you are to base your meals around the following foods:

These types of food combine well with the keto diet:

Meat: *steak, ham, chicken, sausage, bacon, and turkey*
Fatty fish: *trout, tuna, mackerel, and salmon*
Eggs: *omega-3 whole eggs*
Butter and cream: *dairy products of grass-fed animals*
Cheese: *unprocessed cheddar, cream, goat, blue or mozzarella*
Nuts and seeds: *almonds, flax seeds, walnuts, and pumpkin seeds*
Healthy oils: *extra virgin olive oil, coconut and avocado oil*
Avocados: *whole avocado or fresh guacamole*
Low-carb veggies: *greens, tomatoes, peppers, and onions*

In the keto diet, it's recommended to base your meals on whole, one-ingredient types of food.

You should always try to change the mix of your vegetables and meats to reduce the boredom in the diet and increase your nutritional intake of vital chemicals and substances per day. You can have a number of delicious and nutritious meals when following a special keto diet plan, which we are going to present you in this book.

HOW CAN I PREPARE MYSELF FOR THE KETO DIET?

When you decide to go on this high-fat, low-carb diet, you should be aware of the steps that you should take to be a success, feel and be healthy and lose weight in the end.

The keto diet might be difficult to start for some people. Since it's likely to be a step aside from the way you're feeding yourself now. Nowadays a lot of people decide for the keto diet, which puts their body in ketosis. To get into this state, you need to be aware of the following facts.

Firstly, you should limit the carbohydrates intake. Mostly, people tend to think about pure carbohydrates at first. Well, if you go on the keto diet, you should try to get less than 20 grams (0.705 oz) of pure carbohydrates and less than 35 grams (1.234 oz) of carbohydrates daily.

Secondly, you should also limit protein intake because too much protein can cause lower level of ketosis. It is advisable to get between 0.6 g (0.021 oz) and 0.8 g (0.028 oz) of proteins per pound of body mass.

Thirdly, do not worry about fat! On the keto diet, fat is the main energy source - so make sure you eat enough. Remember: the keto diet doesn't presuppose that you lose weight just because of hunger. Nobody is going to starve on this diet.

Fourthly, you should drink a lot of liquid, mainly clean water. It is recommended to drink around 1 gallon (that's 3.8 litres) of water per day. Liquid helps not only to control essential functions of the organism, but also to restrain hunger.

Fifthly, please do not have any snacks in-between the meals!

You will lose weight more effectively and fast when you have less insulin in the blood in a day. Too many snacks during the day can slow down the desired process of losing weight.

And finally, do not forget about exercising.

It is well-known that exercise improves your health and helps to become slim combines with diets. If you want to get the best results on the keto diet, you should have at least 20+ minutes of exercise daily.

Here are some ideas as to what exercise can be good for you. You can take short walks in the morning and in the evening which can control your blood sugar levels.

Another way of exercising is go to the swimming pool twice a week. This will exert a positive effect on your body.

And the last but not least: be careful when choosing food in the supermarket: double check the ingredients of the products on the labels. You often find hidden carbs in food that can seem good for the keto diet.

RECIPES

RECIPES

WHAT YOU CAN HAVE FOR BREAKFAST ON THE KETO DIET

Do you want to feel light and airy? Then the following recipe is just for you. Taco "Keto" will fill your morning with energy; it will give all the necessary elements to your body and help you on the way to a healthier lifestyle.

TACO "KETO"

How long it takes to prepare: 30 minutes
The number of serves: 3

THE INGREDIENTS:

- ♦ 8 oz. of mozzarella cheese
- ♦ 6 large eggs
- ♦ 2 tablespoons of butter
- ♦ 3 slices of bacon
- ♦ A half of avocado
- ♦ 1 oz. of Cheddar cheese
- ♦ Pepper and salt to taste

HOW TO COOK IT:

1. First, you should heat an oven up to 375 °F. Then put the foil on a baking sheet. Spread the bacon on it. Cook the bacon for 20 minutes.

2. While bacon is being cooked, put 3 oz. of mozzarella in a pan. Cook the cheese at medium heat.

3. Wait for the cheese to roast around the edges; it will take about 3 minutes.

4. Use a pair of tongs and a wooden spoon to make a cheese shell for tacos.

5. Do the same with the other pieces of cheese.

6. Cook the eggs in the oil, stirring from time to time. Add salt and pepper.

7. 7. Put the eggs, avocado and bacon in each of the hardened taco casings.

8. Sprinkle the dish with cheddar cheese.

9. Enjoy your meal.

CALORIES PER SERVING:

Calories: 444. Fat: 1.27 oz Protein: 0.91 oz Carbs: 0.08 oz

MORNING OMELET "KETO"

How long it takes to prepare: 15 minutes
The number of serves: 1

THE INGREDIENTS:

- 3 large eggs
- 1 green onion
- 1 oz. of goat cheese
- ¼ onion
- 2 tablespoons of butter
- 2 cups of spinach
- 2 tablespoons of thick cream
- Salt and pepper to taste

HOW TO COOK IT:

1. Cut the onion into long strips and fry these strips in oil until caramelized. Add the spinach to the pan and fry it for a little while.
2. Mix the three eggs, thick cream, and salt and pepper together.
3. Pour the egg mixture into the pan and cook on medium heat.
4. Add a spoonful of green spinach and onions to the omelet and sprinkle with the chopped goat cheese when the edges of the omelet begin to fry.
5. When the top of the omelet is ready, you can serve it. If you like, you can decorate it with onions on top.

CALORIES PER SERVING:

Calories: 621. Fat: 1.94 oz Protein: 1.30 oz Carbs: 4.8

STUFFED AVOCADO

How long it takes to prepare: 15 minutes
The number of serves: 1

THE INGREDIENTS:

- 1 pitted avocado
- 1 tablespoon of butter, salted
- 3 large eggs
- 3 slices of bacon cut into small pieces
- Plus salt and black pepper

HOW TO COOK IT:

1. Clean the avocado pulp out, but you should leave about 1.5 cm.

2. Place a big frying pan at low heat temperature and add butter onto it. Melt the butter. Then break the eggs into the bowl and whisk them well. Add a pinch of salt and pepper.

3. Place bacon on one side of the pan and fry for a couple of minutes. On the other side pour the egg mixture and stir it regularly.

4. Eggs and bacon should be cooked five minutes after adding eggs to the pan.

5. Mix the bacon with scrambled eggs, and then fill the avocado halves with this mixture.

CALORIES PER SERVING:

Calories: 500. Fat: 1.41 oz Protein: 0.88 oz. Carbs: 0.38 oz

VEGETARIAN SCRAMBLE

How long it takes to prepare: 20 minutes
The number of serves: 5

Note! This dish is very easy to cook and you will enjoy eating avocadoes, tomatoes and cheese. This will definitely improve your health and you will definitely feel much better.

THE INGREDIENTS:

- ◆ 1 lb. tofu cheese
- ◆ 3 tablespoons of avocado oil
- ◆ 2 tablespoons of chopped onion
- ◆ 1½ tablespoons of food yeast
- ◆ ½ tablespoons of garlic powder
- ◆ ½ tablespoons of turmeric
- ◆ ½ tablespoons of salt
- ◆ 1 cup of spinach
- ◆ 3 tomatoes
- ◆ 3 oz. vegan Cheddar Cheese

HOW TO COOK IT:

1. Wrap up tofu in a few layers of paper. Squeeze some water softly. Put it aside.
2. In a skillet at medium heat, fry the chopped onion in 1/3 tbsp. of avocado butter until onion is semi-transparent.
3. Place the tofu in the pan and stir it well using a fork.
4. Pour the oil and sprinkle with dry seasoning.
5. Fry tofu at medium heat. Stir from time to time till most of the water has evaporated.
6. Add spinach. Dice the tomatoes and add cheddar cheese.
7. Cook for one minute.
8. Serve this dish hot.

CALORIES PER SERVING:

Calories: 211. Fat: 0.62 oz Protein: 0.35 oz Carbs: 0.17 oz

CHICKEN AND CHEESE QUESADILLA

How long it takes to prepare: 25 minutes
The number of serves: 4

THE INGREDIENTS:

For lozenges:

♦ 6 Eggs

♦ 4 oz. coconut flour

♦ 6 oz. thick cream

♦ ½ tablespoon of Xanthan gum

♦ Pink salt and pepper

♦ 1 tablespoon of Olive oil

For the quesadilla you will need:

♦ 4 oz. of Cheddar cheese, shredded

♦ 8 oz. of Chicken breast cooked

♦ 1 tablespoon of parsley, chopped

HOW TO COOK IT:

1. Mix all the ingredients. Whisk well. Let the dough stand for 10 minutes.

2. Heat the oil in a frying pan at medium heat. Fry the tortillas for 2-3 minutes on each side or until cooked.

3. Put one tortilla, sprinkle with cheese, cover with a lid. Wait until the cheese begins to melt. Then add chopped chicken meat, cheese and cover with a second flat cake.

4. After the cheese has melted, remove the quesadilla from the pan. Cut it into four slices and sprinkle with parsley.

NOTE: If you want to get the best results, you need to use ground coconut flour. Thus, you can prepare thin cakes. Xanthan gum will make the tortilla strong and elastic. Instead of fat cream, you can use almond milk without sugar.

CALORIES PER SERVING:

Calories: 382. Fat: 1.09 oz Protein: 0.81 oz Carbs: 0.08 oz

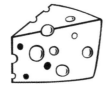

KETO BURGER WITH GUACAMOLE AND EGG

How long it takes to prepare: 15 minutes
The number of serves: 1

If you really love burgers, here's a very good and healthy recipe of a mouthwatering burger. You will need only 15 minutes and then you can enjoy the Keto burger.

THE INGREDIENTS:

- ♦ 5 oz. of ground beef
- ♦ 4 slices of bacon
- ♦ 3 oz. of guacamole
- ♦ 1 egg
- ♦ 1tablespoon of Olive oil
- ♦ ½ tablespoon of Italian seasoning
- ♦ Salt and pepper to taste

HOW TO COOK IT:

1. Mix ground beef with Italian seasoning, salt and pepper in a bowl. Shape a small patty.
2. Put four strips of bacon crosswise on a cutting board, cutlet on top. Then wrap bacon around it.
3. Warm up 1/2 tablespoons of olive oil in a frying pan at medium heat.
4. Add the cutlet in bacon. Fry for three minutes on each side.
5. Add the remaining 1/2 tablespoons of oil to the pan and fry the egg.
6. Put a guacamole, a fried egg on a cutlet, and season with salt and pepper.
7. Cut in half and serve the dish.

CALORIES PER SERVING:

Calories: 443. Fat: 1.16 oz Protein: 1.15oz Carbs: 0.08 oz

NEAPOLITAN FATTY BOMBS

How long it takes to prepare: 25 minutes
The number of serves: 24

THE INGREDIENTS:

- ♦ ½ cup butter
- ♦ ½ cup coconut oil
- ♦ ½ cup sour cream
- ♦ ½ cup cream cheese
- ♦ 2 tablespoons of Erythritol
- ♦ 25 drops of liquid stevia
- ♦ 2 tablespoons of cocoa powder
- ♦ 1 tablespoon of vanilla extract
- ♦ 2 medium-sized strawberries

HOW TO COOK IT:

1. Mix all the ingredients in a blender (cocoa powder, vanilla and strawberry do not add at this stage).

2. Divide the mixture into three bowls. Add cocoa powder to the first bowl, vanilla to another, and strawberries to the third one.

3. Pour the chocolate mixture into the mold. Place it in the freezer for 30 minutes. Do the same with the others.

4. Now put into the fridge to freeze for at least 1 hour.

CALORIES PER SERVING:

Calories: 102. Fat: 0.92 oz. Protein: 0.035 oz. Carbs: 0.017 oz

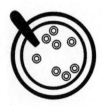

ALMOND CHOCOLATE COCONUT FAT BOMBS

How long it takes to prepare: 20 minutes
The number of serves: 12

THE INGREDIENTS:

♦ 1 cup of coconut chips

♦ 3 tablespoons of fat coconut milk

♦ 3 tablespoons of coconut oil

♦ ½ tablespoon of vanilla extract

♦ 4 oz. of chocolate chips, without sugar

♦ a pinch of salt

♦ 2 oz. of keto-friendly sweetener

♦ 24 almonds

HOW TO COOK IT:

1. Put 2 tablespoons of melted coconut oil, coconut milk, sweetener, coconut chips, vanilla extract and salt into a bowl.

2. Separate the mixture into 12 servings.

3. Place them on a baking sheet with parchment paper.

4. Put them in the freezer for 5 minutes, and then put on each fat bomb 2 almonds.

5. Melt the chocolate chips together with 2 teaspoons of coconut oil in the microwave.

6. Take the bombs out of the freezer, and pour in the chocolate mixture.

CALORIES PER SERVING:

Calories: 92. Fat: 0.32 oz. Protein: 0.075 oz. Carbs: 0.05 oz.

SPICY FAT BOMBS

How long it takes to prepare: 20 minutes
The number of serves: 12

THE INGREDIENTS:

- ◆ 6 MCT powder, scoops
- ◆ 10 liquid stevia, drops
- ◆ 1 tablespoon of turmeric
- ◆ 1 tablespoon of black sesame seeds
- ◆ a pinch of Chinese 5 Spice Blend
- ◆ a pinch of black pepper
- ◆ ½ tablespoon of Cinnamon
- ◆ 2½ fl. oz. warm water

HOW TO COOK IT:

1. Mix all the dry ingredients in a small bowl.
2. Add warm water and mix until it becomes smooth.
3. Spread the mixture evenly over 12 silicone molds, about one tablespoon on each one.
4. Put them in the fridge so that the fat bombs become well frozen.
5. You should always keep them frozen, otherwise they will quickly melt.

CALORIES PER SERVING:

Calories: 81. Fat: 0.28 oz. Protein: 0.03 oz. Carbs: 0.05 oz

COFFEE FAT BOMBS

How long it takes to prepare: 35 minutes
The number of serves: 12

THE INGREDIENTS:

- ◆ 4 oz. of butter
- ◆ 2 oz. of ghee butter (melted)
- ◆ 2 oz. of thick cream
- ◆ 1 tablespoon of milk
- ◆ double espresso
- ◆ 2 oz. of Keto-friendly sweetener
- ◆ 1 tablespoon of vanilla extract
- ◆ a pinch of salt

HOW TO COOK IT:

1. Add the ingredients to a small food processor and whip at high speed until airy.
2. Add sweetener.
3. Pour into molds and cool in the fridge for 30 minutes.

CALORIES PER SERVING:

Calories: 61. Fat: 0.17 oz. Protein: 0.035 oz. Carbs: 0.035 oz

ALMOND COCONUT FAT BOMBS

How long it takes to prepare: 25 minutes
The number of serves: 10

THE INGREDIENTS:

- 2 fl. oz. almond oil
- 2 fl. oz coconut oil
- 2 tablespoon of cocoa powder
- 2 fl. oz erythritol

HOW TO COOK IT:

1. Mix almond and coconut oil.

2. Heat the mixture in the microwave for 30-45 seconds.

3. Mix it until you get a homogeneous mass. Add erythritol and cocoa powder, and mix it well.

4. Pour the mass into mini-cupcake molds and refrigerate.

CALORIES PER SERVING:

Calories: 89. Fat: 0.32 oz. Protein: 0.052 oz. Carbs: 0.035 oz.

PUMPKIN FAT SPICE BOMBS

How long it takes to prepare: 15 minutes
The number of serves: 9

THE INGREDIENTS:

- ◆ 8 oz. raw cashews
- ◆ 4 oz. raw macadamia nuts
- ◆ 4 oz. coconut chips
- ◆ 3 fl. oz. pumpkin puree
- ◆ 2 tbsp. MCT oils
- ◆ 2 tsp. cinnamon, ground
- ◆ 2 tsp. ginger, ground
- ◆ Avocado oil

HOW TO COOK IT:

1. Put the ingredients in a food processor and mix to form dough.
2. Lightly grease your hands with some oil, e.g. avocado oil.
3. With a spoon, take about 3.5 -4 oz. of the batter into lightly oiled hands and form a ball.
4. Repeat the process (you should form about 9 "bombs" in total).
5. Decorate fat bombs with savory coconut chips.
6. Such fatty bombs can be eaten immediately.

CALORIES PER SERVING:

Calories: 217. Fat: 0.67 oz. Protein: 0.18 oz. Carbs: 0.18 oz.

CHEESE & BACON FAT BOMBS

How long it takes to prepare: 25 minutes
The number of serves: 20

THE INGREDIENTS:

- 8 oz. of Mozzarella cheese
- 4 tablespoons of almond flour
- 4 tablespoons of butter, melted
- 3 tablespoons of Psyllium powder
- 1 egg
- a pinch of salt
- 1 tablespoon of black pepper
- 1/8 tablespoon of garlic powder
- 1/8 tablespoon of onion powder
- 20 slices of bacon
- 1 cup of oil or lard

HOW TO COOK IT:

1. Heat the cheese for 45-60 seconds in a microwave.
2. Heat the butter in the microwave for 15-20 seconds until completely melted
3. Mix it with cheese and egg.
4. Add Psyllium husks, almond flour and spices. Mix again and lay out the dough in a rectangular form.
5. Fill the rectangle with the rest of the cheese and fold it in half (horizontally), then in half (vertically).
6. Trim the edges and form a rectangle. Cut 20 square pieces.
7. 7. Wrap each piece of dough with a piece of bacon, using toothpicks to fasten it.
8. 7. Put each piece in boiling oil and cook for 1-3 minutes.

CALORIES PER SERVING:

Calories: 93. Fat: 0.28 oz. Protein: 0.17 oz. Carbs: 0.035 oz.

VEGETABLE SALAD WITH BACON & CHEESE

How long it takes to prepare: 15 minutes
The number of serves: 6

THE INGREDIENTS:

- ◆ 4 oz. lettuce
- ◆ 3 oz. spinach
- ◆ 2 oz. curly cabbage
- ◆ 6 slices of cooked bacon
- ◆ 12 pieces of grape tomato
- ◆ 1 avocado, peeled and sliced
- ◆ 2 oz. of blue cheese
- ◆ 3 tablespoons of sour cream
- ◆ 2 ½ tablespoons of mayo

HOW TO COOK IT:

1. Mix sour cream with mayonnaise in a small bowl.
2. Mix it with the blue cheese and set aside.
3. In a large salad bowl, mix the remaining ingredients.
4. Spread the salad into portions and place the blue cheese dressing on top.

CALORIES PER SERVING:

Calories: 183. Fat: 0.56 oz. Protein: 0.22 oz. Carbs: 0.088 oz.

SALAD WITH CHICKEN BREAST & GREENS

How long it takes to prepare: 40 minutes
The number of serves: 2

THE INGREDIENTS:

- 2 tablespoons of pesto sauce
- 2 fl. oz. of balsamic vinegar
- 1 tablespoon of Olive oil
- 6 oz. of chicken breast
- 4 cup of spring greens
- 1 oz. of fresh mozzarella
- ¼ avocado, diced
- 6 cherry tomatoes
- 1 tablespoon of fresh basil

HOW TO COOK IT:

1. Cook the marinade by mixing pesto, balsamic vinegar and olive oil.

2. Put aside a portion of the marinade for the salad.

3. Pour the remaining portion into chicken breast. Refrigerate marinate for at least 20 minutes.

4. Cook the salad. Start with greens, and then add fresh mozzarella, avocado and tomatoes.

5. Once the chicken is pickled, heat the medium-sized griddle, and then add a little olive oil.

6. Fry each side of the breast for 10 minutes.

7. 7. Slice the chicken breast and put in previously prepared salad.

8. Pour the remaining balsamic pesto and add some chopped fresh basil.

CALORIES PER SERVING:

Calories: 306. Fat: 0.56 oz. Protein: 0.88 oz. Carbs: 0.23 oz

WHAT YOU CAN HAVE FOR LUNCH ON THE KETO DIET

Here we are presenting to you the best recipes to enhance your keto experience. The dishes are varied so everyone can find the one for themselves. And remember, you are on the way to a healthier and happier life.

KETO CHICKEN NUGGETS

How long it takes to prepare: 30 minutes
The number of serves: 2

THE INGREDIENTS:

- 1 oz. whipped egg whites
- 1 oz. chicken breast cooked and minced beforehand
- ½ oz. coconut flour
- ½ tablespoon baking powder
- 1 fl. oz. of olive oil
- ½ oz. butter
- 1 oz. of 40%-fat cream
- salt, pepper, a pinch of garlic powder

HOW TO COOK IT:

1. Add the coconut flour to the chicken meat with, and then add baking powder. This mixture should be very dry.

2. Add butter and then mix it again. Add whipped egg whites and mix until it is smooth.

3. Pour the olive oil into a small pan. Spread the chicken-egg mixture in small pieces and fry them for approximately one minute on each side.

4. Serve the dish with whipped cream.

CALORIES PER SERVING:

Calories: 136. Fat: 1.45 oz. Protein: 0.32 oz. Carbs: 0.07 oz.

KETO CHAMPIGNON BURGER

How long it takes to prepare: 20 minutes
The number of serves: 4

THE INGREDIENTS:

- 2 big champignons
- 2 tablespoons of olive oil
- 1 tablespoon of balsamic vinegar
- 2 slices of bacon
- 4 oz. of ground beef
- ½ tablespoon of garlic powder
- ½ tablespoon of onion powder
- ½ tablespoon of Worcestershire Sauce
- 1 slice of cheddar cheese
- 1 slice of tomato
- 2 oz. of mixed greens
- 1 tablespoon of low-sugar ketchup
- Salt and pepper

HOW TO COOK IT:

1. Put the mushroom caps in a bowl. Add olive oil, balsamic vinegar and salt and pepper. Marinate the mushrooms for at least half an hour.

2. Cook the bacon in a frying pan over medium heat until it gets crisp. Then set aside.

3. Pre-heat the oven to 270 °F degrees. Mix in a bowl ground beef, garlic and onion powder, Worcestershire sauce, and salt and pepper.

4. Shape the patties for burgers.

5. Put the caps of champignons and cutlets on the grill, and cook for about 4 minutes on each side until they are soft. At the last minute, put cheese on the cutlets so that it melts.

6. Put together the hamburger with bacon and the stuffing between the mushroom caps.

CALORIES PER SERVING:

Calories: 771. Fat: 2.36 oz. Protein: 1.31 oz. Carbs: 0.14 oz

KETO BEEF SOUP

How long it takes to prepare: 40 minutes
The number of serves: 8

THE INGREDIENTS:

- 1 lb. of ground beef
- 5 slices of bacon
- 1 tablespoon of olive oil
- 1 tablespoon of minced garlic
- 1 cup of chopped celery
- 1½ cup of bone broth
- 1 cup of shredded cheddar
- 2 fl. oz. fat whipped cream
- 2 tsp. Psyllium powder
- 4 oz. of shredded cheddar cheese
- ½ oz. of chopped green onions
- ½ cup of sour cream

HOW TO COOK IT:

1. Fry the bacon over medium heat. Place it on a piece of paper towels to get rid of unnecessary fat. Then, cut it into pieces.

2. Fry the ground beef at medium heat. After doing so, drain the fat and put the minced meat to a bowl.

3. In the same pan, melt butter over medium heat. Add chopped garlic and fry until fragrant.

4. Add the celery and cook for about 5 minutes until slightly softened.

5. Put the ground beef in the pan. Add beef broth, cheddar, and fat whipped cream, sautéed celery with garlic, bacon, salt and pepper. Cook for 20 minutes, stirring from time to time.

6. To get the desired thickness of the mixture, you should add Psyllium powder.

7. 7. Pour into portions and add a side dish in the form of cheese, green onions and sour cream (if you like).

CALORIES PER SERVING:

Calories: 349. Fat: 0.95 oz. Protein: 0.81 oz. Carbs: 0.11 oz

KETO CHEESEBURGER WITH BACON

How long it takes to prepare: 40 minutes
The number of serves: 2

THE INGREDIENTS:

For the dough:

- ◆ 8 oz. of shredded mozzarella,
- ◆ 4 oz. of almond flour
- ◆ 1 tablespoon of cream cheese

For the filling:

- ◆ 5 oz. of ground beef
- ◆ 1 slice of cheddar cheese, cut into quarters
- ◆ 1 tablespoon of mustard
- ◆ 4 slices of bacon
- ◆ 1 whisked egg
- ◆ 1 tablespoon of sesame
- ◆ 1 tablespoon of olive oil

HOW TO COOK IT:

1. Pre-heat the oven to around 420 °F degrees.
2. Mix mozzarella, almond flour and cream cheese in a bowl.
3. Heat the mix in the microwave for one minute. Then mix again and put it in the microwave again for one minute.
4. Shape two patties from ground beef. Put on the cutting board four slices of bacon crosswise, then cutlet on top, then cheddar slices, the second cutlet, and then wrap everything in the bacon.
5. Heat the olive oil in a frying pan over medium heat. Put the patties in bacon and fry them for three minutes turning them on each side.
6. Roll the dough between two sheets of parchment paper.

7. Take away the top layer and put mustard in the center of the dough. On top, put the patty in bacon and wrap the dough.

8. Put the burger in the oven, coat with beaten egg, and sprinkle with sesame seeds and bake for around 20 minutes or until golden brown.

CALORIES PER SERVING:

Calories: 411. Fat: 1.13 oz. Protein: 0.95 oz. Carbs: 0.11 oz.

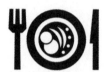

SPICY KETO SOUP + MUSHROOMS

How long it takes to prepare: 40 minutes
The number of serves: 4

THE INGREDIENTS:

- 1 tablespoon of olive oil
- 1 sliced onion (thinly sliced)
- 1 tablespoon of freshly grated ginger
- 3 garlic cloves
- 1 tablespoon of chili
- 1 tablespoon of fish sauce
- 2 fl. oz. of soy sauce
- 2 fl. oz. of rice vinegar
- 4 oz. of mushrooms
- 4 hard boiled eggs
- 2-3 packets of shirataki noodles
- 5 cups of bone broth

HOW TO COOK IT:

1. Pour oil into a saucepan and put on medium heat.
2. Add the onion and cook for 2-3 minutes until it is soft.
3. Add the other ingredients to the pan (Note! Eggs and noodles will be added later). Cook over low heat for 20 minutes.
4. Rinse the noodles under cold water.
5. Add seasoning to the broth and mix with noodles.
6. Pour the broth into portions.
7. Add hard-boiled eggs, chopped chicken, sesame seeds, chopped onions and chili sauce.

CALORIES PER SERVING:

Calories: 103. Fat: 0.46oz. Protein: 0.42 oz. Carbs: 0.25 oz.

GREEK KETO MOUSSAKA

How long it takes to prepare: 40 minutes
The number of serves: 4

THE INGREDIENTS:

For the filling:

♦ ½ of a chopped eggplant

♦ 10 oz. of minced chicken

♦ 3 tablespoons of Marinara sauce

♦ 1 minced garlic

♦ ½ chopped onion

♦ 1 tablespoon of dried oregano

♦ 1 tablespoon of paprika

♦ ½ tablespoon of ground cinnamon

♦ 2 tablespoons of olive oil

For the sauce:

♦ 3 tablespoons of the thick cream

♦ 3 tablespoons of cream cheese

♦ 3 oz. of crushed cheddar cheese

♦ 1 minced garlic

HOW TO COOK IT:

1. Lay out a foil baking sheet.
2. Cut the eggplants.
3. Put the eggplants on the baking sheet and pour olive oil.
4. Bake the eggplants for five minutes.
5. Heat olive oil in a frying pan, add chopped onion, chopped garlic and fry until soft.
6. Add chopped chicken, and fry until the meat is cooked.
7. Add the marinara sauce, mix and cook for another 3 minutes.

8. Mix half of the crushed cheddar cheese, cream cheese, thick cream, garlic and salt in a saucepan.

9. Cook on low heat until the cheese is melted and the sauce becomes thick.

10. Preheat oven to 400 °F degrees. Put the pieces of fried eggplant on the baking sheet, top the chicken mixture, and pour the sauce, then sprinkle with the grated cheese and bake this dish for 20 min.

11. Let the dish stand for 5 minutes before serving.

CALORIES PER SERVING:

Calories: 358. Fat: 1.02 oz. Protein: 0.71 oz. Carbs: 0.14 oz.

ALMOND PANCAKES WITH SHRIMP AND CHEESE

How long it takes to prepare: 20 minutes
The number of serves: 8

THE INGREDIENTS:

- ◆ 1 lb. of shrimp cooked and chopped
- ◆ 2 oz. of almond flour
- ◆ 1 whisked egg
- ◆ 2 oz. of mozzarella, shredded
- ◆ 3 tablespoons of Parmesan cheese, grated
- ◆ 1 tablespoon of fresh dill, chopped
- ◆ 1½ tablespoons of olive or coconut oil
- ◆ Salt and pepper

HOW TO COOK IT:

1. Mix the shrimp, egg, almond flour, cheese, dill in a bowl until smooth.
2. Using a tablespoon, shape pancakes. The size of each one depends on your choice.
3. Heat the oil in a pan over medium heat and fry pancakes for 3-4 minutes on each side.
4. Put on a plate and serve with herbs.

CALORIES PER SERVING:

Calories: 364. Fat: 0.74 oz. Protein: 1.45 oz. Carbs: 0.07 oz.

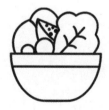

KETO MINI PIZZA

How long it takes to prepare: 20 minutes
The number of serves: 4

THE INGREDIENTS:

- ♦ 1 oz. of keto mayo
- ♦ 1 tablespoon of raw eggs
- ♦ 2 tablespoons of coconut oil, melted
- ♦ 2 tablespoons of almond flour
- ♦ 1 tablespoon of coconut flour
- ♦ ½ tablespoon of Psyllium powder
- ♦ a pinch of baking powder and baking soda

HOW TO COOK IT:

1. Heat the oven to 400 °F degrees.
2. Mix all the ingredients to make dough. There shouldn't be any lumps in it.
3. Let the dough stand for about 5 minutes.
4. Divide the dough into 3-4 small balls.
5. Lay out a baking sheet with parchment paper. Put the balls on the parchment and press down on them to make small pizzas.
6. Put the stuffing on the raw dough and bake the pizza for 7-9 minutes.

CALORIES PER SERVING:

Calories: 112. Fat: 0.99 oz. Protein: 0.14 oz. Carbs: 0.07 oz.

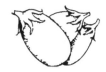

BAKED EGGS WITH HAM AND ASPARAGUS

How long it takes to prepare: 20 minutes
The number of serves: 2

THE INGREDIENTS:

- ♦ 6 Eggs
- ♦ 6 slices of Italian ham
- ♦ 8 oz. of asparagus
- ♦ A few sprigs of fresh marjoram
- ♦ 1 tablespoon of butter

HOW TO COOK IT:

1. Heat the oven to 350°F degrees.
2. Grease the muffin tray.
3. Lay the ham on the tray.
4. Add a few sprigs of marjoram.
5. Pour 1 egg into each form.
6. Put in the oven and bake for 10 - 12 minutes.
7. 7. Pull out and allow it to cool for a few minutes.
8. Steam the asparagus, and then season it with butter.
9. Put all the ingredients on a plate and bon appétit!

CALORIES PER SERVING:

Calories: 424. Fat: 1.16 oz. Protein: 1.06 oz. Carbs: 0.09 oz.

EGGPLANT KETO CHIPS

How long it takes to prepare: 25 minutes
The number of serves: 4

THE INGREDIENTS:

- ◆ 2 fl. oz. of olive oil
- ◆ 1 large eggplant
- ◆ 1 tablespoon of garlic powder
- ◆ ½ tablespoon of dry basil
- ◆ ½ tablespoon of dried oregano
- ◆ 2 tablespoons of parmesan cheese
- ◆ salt and pepper

HOW TO COOK IT:

1. Preheat the oven to 350 °F degrees.
2. Add 1/4 cup of olive oil and dried spices to a small bowl.
3. Roll the sliced eggplant in oil and spices.
4. Place it on a baking sheet.
5. Bake it for about 15-20 minutes, until the chips are evenly fried. Turn them over several times while cooking.
6. Remove from the oven and sprinkle with Parmesan cheese.

CALORIES PER SERVING:

Calories: 60. Fat: 0.18 oz. Protein: 0.07oz. Carbs: 0.03 oz.

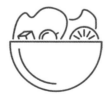

CHEESE KETO STICKS

How long it takes to prepare: 20 minutes
The number of serves: 3

THE INGREDIENTS:

- ◆ 3 Mozzarella cheese sticks (cut in half)
- ◆ 4 oz. of almond flour
- ◆ 1 tablespoon of Italian seasoning mixes
- ◆ 2 tablespoons of grated parmesan cheese
- ◆ 1 big egg
- ◆ salt, to taste
- ◆ 2 tablespoons of coconut oil
- ◆ 1 tablespoon of Chopped parsley

HOW TO COOK IT:

1. Put the cheese in the freezer for 12 hours. It should harden up.
2. Add coconut oil to a medium-sized cast iron skillet.
3. Heat it over low to medium heat.
4. Break the egg into a shallow bowl and whisk well.
5. In a separate bowl, mix the almond flour, parmesan cheese and seasonings.
6. Roll cheese sticks in an egg, then dry breading.
7. 7. Put on a wire rack and bake until golden brown on all sides for about 1-
8. 2 minutes.
9. Place chopsticks on paper towels to soak up the oil.
10. Serve with low-carb marinara sauce and parsley.

CALORIES PER SERVING:

Calories: 436. Fat: 1.38 oz. Protein: 0.71 oz. Carbs: 0.18 oz.

WHAT YOU CAN HAVE FOR DINNER ON THE KETO DIET

BAKED HALIBUT CHEESE BREAD

How long it takes to prepare: 25 minutes
The number of serves: 6

THE INGREDIENTS:

- ◆ 2 lb. of halibut (about 6 fillets)
- ◆ 1 tablespoon of butter
- ◆ 3 tablespoons of grated parmesan cheese
- ◆ 1 tablespoon of bread crumbs
- ◆ 2 tablespoons of garlic powder
- ◆ 1 tablespoon of dried parsley
- ◆ salt and pepper

HOW TO COOK IT:

1. Pre-heat the oven to 400°F degrees.
2. Mix everything thoroughly in a bowl.
3. Dry the fish fillets with a paper towel.
4. Place each fish fillet on a greased buttered parchment tray.
5. Spread the cheese mixture into small pieces of fish so that it covers the top.
6. Bake the fish for around 12 minutes.
7. Turn up the heat for 2–3 minutes until the top gets golden brown.
8. Check if it is cooked well with a fork.

CALORIES PER SERVING:

Calories: 330. Fat: 1.05 oz. Protein: 0.45 oz. Carbs: 0.07 oz.

CHICKEN LEGS

How long it takes to prepare: 35 minutes
The number of serves: 6

THE INGREDIENTS:

- ♦ 2 whole chicken legs
- ♦ 4 fl. oz. fatty Greek yogurt
- ♦ 2 tablespoons of olive oil
- ♦ ½ tablespoon of cumin
- ♦ ½ tablespoon of turmeric
- ♦ ½ tablespoon of coriander
- ♦ 1/4 tablespoon of cardamom
- ♦ ½ tablespoon of cayenne pepper
- ♦ 1 tablespoon of paprika
- ♦ Pinch of Nutmeg
- ♦ 1 minced garlic clove
- ♦ ½ tablespoon of fresh ginger
- ♦ 2 tablespoons of lime juice
- ♦ salt and pepper

HOW TO COOK IT:

1. Heat olive oil in a frying pan over medium heat.
2. Add the spices - cumin, turmeric, coriander, cardamom, cayenne pepper, paprika and a pinch of nutmeg.
3. Heat the spices, then remove from heat and cool.
4. Mix in a bowl yogurt with spiced oil, lime juice, ginger, chopped garlic, salt and pepper.
5. Make four deep cuts on each leg and pour the spicy yogurt inside.
6. Cover and put in the fridge for 6 hours.

7. Lubricate the rack for frying olive oil and place on a baking sheet.

8. Put the chicken on the rack and fry for 5 minutes on each side.

9. Set the oven to 360°F degrees and continue cooking for 25 minutes.

CALORIES PER SERVING:

Calories: 372. Fat: 0.99 oz. Protein: 1.06 oz. Carbs: 0.07 oz.

BAKED EGGPLANT WITH CHEESE

How long it takes to prepare: 75 minutes
The number of serves: 4

THE INGREDIENTS:

- ◆ 1 big eggplant, sliced
- ◆ 1 big egg
- ◆ ½ cup of parmesan cheese, grated
- ◆ ¼ cup of pork dough
- ◆ ½ tablespoon of Italian seasoning
- ◆ 1 cup of low-sugar tomato sauce
- ◆ ½ cup of mozzarella, shredded
- ◆ 4 tablespoons of butter

HOW TO COOK IT:

1. Pre-heat the oven to 400 °F degrees.

2. Put the sliced eggplant on a baking sheet with a paper towel around and sprinkle with salt on both sides of it.

3. Let it stand for at least 30 minutes so that all the water leaves the eggplant.

4. Mix the chopped pork cracklings, parmesan cheese and Italian seasoning in a shallow dish.

5. In a separate small plate, beat an egg.

6. Melt the butter and grease the baking dish with it.

7. Dip each piece of eggplant in a beaten egg.

8. Then put it in a mixture of parmesan and cracklings, covering each side with crumbs.

9. Place the eggplants in a baking dish and bake for 20 minutes.

10. Turn the eggplant slices over and bake for another 20 minutes or until golden brown.

11. Top with tomato sauce and sprinkle with chopped mozzarella.

12. Put it back to the oven for another 5 minutes.

CALORIES PER SERVING:

Calories: 376. Fat: 0.99 oz. Protein: 0.67 oz. Carbs: 0.25 oz.

SHRIMP AND ZUCCHINI WITH ALFREDO SAUCE

How long it takes to prepare: 20 minutes
The number of serves: 6

THE INGREDIENTS:

- ♦ 8 oz. of shrimp, peeled
- ♦ 2 tablespoons of butter
- ♦ ½ tablespoon of Minced garlic
- ♦ 1 tablespoon of Fresh lemon juice
- ♦ 2 Zucchini
- ♦ 2 oz. of heavy cream
- ♦ 3 oz. of parmesan cheese
- ♦ salt and pepper

HOW TO COOK IT:

1. Make zucchini noodles with a scoop.
2. Heat the butter in a frying pan.
3. Add the chopped garlic, red pepper and fry for 1 minute, stirring all the time.
4. Add shrimp and simmer for about 3 minutes.
5. Add salt and pepper, remove from pan and set aside.
6. Add heavy cream into the same pan, lemon juice, parmesan, and cook for 2 minutes.
7. 7. Add zucchini noodles and cook them for another 2 minutes.
8. Put the shrimp back in the pan and mix well.
9. If necessary, add salt and pepper, garnish with parmesan and chopped parsley and serve immediately.

CALORIES PER SERVING:

Calories: 404. Fat: 0.99 oz. Protein: 1.13 oz. Carbs: 0.18 oz.

CHICKEN BREASTS IN A GARLIC SAUCE

How long it takes to prepare: 35 minutes
The number of serves: 4

THE INGREDIENTS:

For chicken:

♦ 2 chicken breasts

♦ 1 tablespoon of lemon juice

♦ 1/4 tablespoon of chili powder

♦ 1 tablespoon of fresh ginger, grated

♦ 1 minced garlic

♦ ½ tablespoon of coriander powder

♦ ½ tablespoon of turmeric

♦ 1 oz. of butter

For the sauce:

♦ 4 oz. heavy cream

♦ 3 tablespoons of crushed tomatoes

♦ 4 fl. oz. Chicken broth

♦ 1 onion, diced

♦ 1 garlic clove, minced

♦ 1/4 tablespoon of chili powder

♦ 1 tablespoon of fresh ginger

♦ 1/4 tablespoon of cinnamon

HOW TO COOK IT:

1. Cut the chicken breasts into small pieces.

2. Mix them with lemon juice, chili powder, grated ginger, chopped garlic, coriander powder, turmeric, salt and pepper.

3. Heat two tablespoons of butter in a frying pan over medium heat, then add the onions and garlic, and simmer for 2 minutes.

4. Add chicken pieces and cook for 4-5 minutes.

5. When the chicken gets white, you should add heavy cream, chopped tomatoes, seasoning and mix well.

6. Bring to a boil, then reduce the heat to minimum, cover and simmer for 6-7 minutes.

7. If you'd like sauce thicker - remove the lid and simmer it to the desired consistency.

8. Serve with steamed broccoli or any other low-carb product to your taste.

CALORIES PER SERVING:

Calories: 319. Fat: 0.74 oz. Protein: 0.95 oz. Carbs: 0.14 oz.

SALMON FILLET

How long it takes to prepare: 25 minutes
The number of serves: 3

THE INGREDIENTS:

- 2 tablespoons of olive oil
- 3 salmon fillets
- 2 garlic cloves, minced
- 1 cup of heavy whipped cream
- 1 oz. cream cheese
- 2 tablespoons of capers
- 1 tablespoon of lemon juice
- 2 tablespoons of fresh dill
- 2 tablespoons of Parmesan cheese, grated

HOW TO COOK IT:

1. Put a frying pan over medium heat.
2. Heat the olive oil. When the pan gets hot, add salmon fillet.
3. Fry each side for about five minutes.
4. When the salmon is ready, take it away from the pan.
5. In the same pan, roast the chopped garlic over medium heat.
6. Add thick cream, cream cheese, lemon juice and capers.
7. Bring the mixture to light boiling.
8. As soon as the sauce starts to het thicker, put the salmon back in the pan and cover it with creamy sauce.
9. Reduce the heat to medium-low.
10. Garnish with fresh dill and grated Parmesan cheese.

CALORIES PER SERVING:

Calories: 494. Fat: 1.09 oz. Protein: 1.87 oz. Carbs: 0.09 oz

BEEF CASSEROLE WITH CABBAGE AND CHEESE

How long it takes to prepare: 45 minutes
The number of serves: 8

THE INGREDIENTS:

- ♦ 2 lb. of cauliflower
- ♦ 8 oz. of cream cheese
- ♦ 1 lb. of ground beef
- ♦ ½ onion, diced
- ♦ 1 tablespoon of Worcestershire Sauce
- ♦ 1 cup Shredded cracklings
- ♦ 1 egg
- ♦ 2 cup of cheddar cheese, grated
- ♦ 5 oz. of bacon
- ♦ salt and pepper

HOW TO COOK IT:

1. Cut the bacon into pieces.
2. Fry it in a frying pan.
3. Put it on a paper towel to absorb excess fat.
4. Remove most of the fat from the pan. Leave only a few tablespoons.
5. Fry the onions in bacon fat until it is golden brown.
6. Add ground beef and fry well.
7. Add the Worcestershire sauce and seasonings.
8. In a separate bowl, mix the cabbage and cream cheese.
9. Whisk everything together using a hand mixer.
10. Add chopped bacon and egg to beef mixture and mix well.
11. Place the ground beef on the bottom of the baking dish, and put the cauliflower puree on top.

12. Sprinkle casserole with chopped cheddar cheese and bacon.

13. Bake at 400 °F for 30 minutes.

CALORIES PER SERVING:

Calories: 443. Fat: 1.23 oz. Protein: 0.85 oz. Carbs: 0.19 oz.

CREAMY SPINACH

How long it takes to prepare: 30 minutes
The number of serves: 4

THE INGREDIENTS:

- ♦ 2 tablespoons of butter
- ♦ 2 tablespoons of olive oil
- ♦ 1 onion, diced
- ♦ 2 garlic cloves, minced
- ♦ 9 oz. of fresh spinach
- ♦ 2 fl. oz. of cream cheese
- ♦ 2 fl. oz. of heavy cream

HOW TO COOK IT:

1. Heat the cream and olive oil in a frying pan at medium-high heat.
2. Add garlic and onions.
3. Stir continuously for 2-3 minutes until soft.
4. Add the spinach and fry until it withers.
5. Return the spinach to the pan, season with pepper and salt, and add the heavy cream.
6. Cook until bubbles in the cream.
7. 7. Mix with cream cheese until it is completely melted.
8. Remove from heat and serve.

CALORIES PER SERVING:

Calories: 277. Fat: 0.74 oz. Protein: 0.31 oz. Carbs: 0.25 oz.

FRIED COD WITH TOMATO SAUCE

How long it takes to prepare: 30 minutes
The number of serves: 4

THE INGREDIENTS:

A fish:

- ◆ 1 lb. (4 fillets) Cod
- ◆ 1 tablespoon of butter
- ◆ 1 tablespoon of olive oil
- ◆ Salt and pepper

Tomato sauce:

- ◆ 3 big egg yolks
- ◆ 3 tablespoons of warm water
- ◆ 8 oz. butter
- ◆ 2 tablespoons of tomato paste
- ◆ 2 tablespoons of fresh lemon juice

HOW TO COOK IT:

A fish:

1. Season the fillets on both sides. You should add the salt at the last minute before cooking in order not to burn the fish.

2. Pour olive oil over the lower part of the anti-grate pan. Turn on the medium heat.

3. Add butter. When the fillets start to sizzle, add cod fillet. Fry for two or three minutes, then turn them over to the other side.

4. Tilt the pan, collect the oil with a spoon and dip the fish in it. Continue cooking for another two or three minutes.

Tomato sauce:

1. Melt the butter.

2. Boil egg yolks and warm water (1 tablespoon of water for each egg yolk) for two minutes until thick and creamy.

3. When the yolks have reached the desired consistency, remove them from the heat. Then start to beat them, slowly adding butter. Beat them until smooth.

4. Season with salt and pepper.

5. Add tomato paste and mix.

6. Add lemon juice and adjust the consistency with warm water to slightly dilute the sauce.

CALORIES PER SERVING:

Calories: 589. Fat: 1.98 oz. Protein: 0.71 oz. Carbs: 0.07 oz.

BRAISED BEEF IN ORANGE SAUCE

How long it takes to prepare: 120 minutes
The number of serves: 6

THE INGREDIENTS:

- ◆ 2 lb. Beef
- ◆ 3 cups Beef broth
- ◆ 3 tablespoons of coconut oil
- ◆ 1 Onion
- ◆ Peel and juice of one orange
- ◆ 2 tablespoons of apple vinegar
- ◆ 1 tablespoon of fresh thyme
- ◆ 2½ tablespoons of garlic, chopped
- ◆ 2 tablespoons of ground cinnamon
- ◆ 2 tablespoons of Erythritol
- ◆ 1 tablespoon of soy sauce
- ◆ Herbs: rosemary, sage, bay leaf, salt, pepper

HOW TO COOK IT:

1. Cut vegetables and meat into cubes. Squeeze orange juice and rub it in zest.
2. Heat coconut oil in a cast iron skillet.
3. Add seasoned meat to the pan in batches.
4. Fry it until brown and remove from the pan.
5. When the beef is ready, add vegetables to the pan. Cook them for 1-2 minutes.
6. Add orange juice and then put all the other ingredients in the pan, with the exception of rosemary, sage and thyme.
7. 7. Cook for 30 seconds, and then add all other ingredients.

8. Stew for 3 hours.

9. Open up the pan and add the spices. Cook it for 1-2 hours.

CALORIES PER SERVING:

Calories: 337. Fat: 0.49 oz. Protein: 1.48 oz. Carbs: 0.18 oz.

MEATLOAF

How long it takes to prepare: 70 minutes
The number of serves: 6

THE INGREDIENTS:

- 1 lb. ground beef
- ½ tablespoon of garlic powder
- ½ tablespoon of cumin
- 6 slices Cheddar cheese
- 2 oz. sliced onions
- 2 oz. green onions, chopped
- ½ cup of spinach
- ¼ cup of mushrooms

HOW TO COOK IT:

1. Mix the meat with salt, pepper, garlic and cumin. Put the stuffing in the form. But leave a place for the filling in the middle.
2. Put cheese on the bottom of the roll.
3. Add onions, spinach and mushrooms.
4. Cover meat with spinach and mushrooms.
5. Bake at 370 °F for one hour.

CALORIES PER SERVING:

Calories: 248. Fat: 0.74 oz. Protein: 0.53 oz. Carbs: 0.07 oz.

KETO CHILI

How long it takes to prepare: 40 minutes
The number of serves: 6

THE INGREDIENTS:

- 2 lb. young beef
- 8 oz. spinach
- 1 cup tomato sauce
- 2 oz. parmesan cheese
- 2 green bell peppers
- 1 onion
- 1 tablespoon of olive oil
- 1 tablespoon of cumin
- 1½ tablespoons of chili powder
- 2 tablespoons of cayenne pepper
- 1 tablespoon of garlic powder
- salt and pepper

HOW TO COOK IT:

1. Slice the onions and peppers. Add salt and pepper. Simmer in olive oil at medium high temperature, stirring from time to time. After the vegetables are ready, reduce the heat to minimum.

2. Fry the beef until brown. Season it with salt, pepper and spices.

3. When the beef is fried, add spinach. Cook for 2-3 minutes, and then mix well.

4. Add tomato sauce, mix well, then reduce the heat to medium-low and cook for 10 minutes.

5. Add Parmesan cheese and mix everything together. Then add the vegetables and mix again. Cook for a few minutes.

CALORIES PER SERVING:

Calories: 404. Fat: 0.95 oz. Protein: 1.09 oz. Carbs: 0.18 oz.

BEEF CROQUETTES WITH SAUSAGE AND CHEESE

How long it takes to prepare: 40 minutes
The number of serves: 12

THE INGREDIENTS:

- ◆ 1 lb. minced beef
- ◆ 1 chorizo sausage
- ◆ 1 tablespoon of chili
- ◆ 1 cup cheddar cheese
- ◆ 8 fl. oz. tomato sauce
- ◆ 3 oz. shredded pork skins
- ◆ 2 eggs
- ◆ 1 tablespoon of cumin

HOW TO COOK IT:

1. Pre-heat oven to 380 °F degrees.
2. Cut the sausage into small pieces, mix well with the beef.
3. Add pork skins, spices, cheese and eggs.
4. Mix everything together until you can shape the meatballs.
5. Place them on a baking sheet with a baking sheet.
6. Bake in the oven for 30-35 minutes.
7. 7. Top with tomato sauce.

CALORIES PER SERVING:

Calories: 142. Fat: 0.42 oz. Protein: 0.25 oz. Carbs: 0.03 oz.

EGGPLANT WITH BACON

How long it takes to prepare: 30 minutes
The number of serves: 6

THE INGREDIENTS:

- 1 lb. bacon
- 1 lb. eggplant
- 1 cup of heavy whipped cream
- 2 tablespoons of butter
- 2 garlic cloves, grated
- 1 tablespoon of white wine
- 1 tablespoon of lemon juice
- 1 cup Parmesan cheese, shredded

HOW TO COOK IT:

1. Slice the bacon and fry it in a large frying pan over medium heat.

2. As soon as the bacon gets crispy, take it out of the pan and place it on a paper towel. Keep all the fat.

3. Peel and slice the eggplant. Cook it in bacon fat until it softens.

4. During the cooking, the eggplant will get all the fat in it.

5. Clean the center of the place and pour 2 tablespoons of oil into it.

6. Stir everything so that the eggplants are covered in melted butter, and then add the grated garlic.

7. 7. Pour a cup of heavy whipped cream into the pan. Then add white wine and lemon juice.

8. Add a cup of shredded Parmesan cheese and mix.

9. Mix everything with about half the bacon.

10. Serve with the remaining bacon, laid out on top. You can also chop fresh basil from above.

CALORIES PER SERVING:

Calories: 564. Fat: 1.80 oz. Protein: 0.56 oz. Carbs: 0.21 oz.

DESSERTS

DESSERTS

Are you a sweet tooth? At the beginning of the book, you might have thought that you would suffer because of the diet – you probably thought that this diet meant no desserts. Don't fall into despair. The Keto diet is the best diet in the world! Here we present desserts which you can enjoy being on the Keto diet and lead a healthy lifestyle.

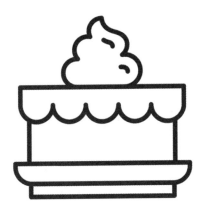

CHEESECAKE KETO-CUPCAKES

How long it takes to prepare: 25 minutes
The number of serves: 12

THE INGREDIENTS:

- 4 oz. of almond flour
- 6 oz. granulated keto sweetener
- 2 oz. butter, melted
- 1 tablespoon of vanilla extract
- 8 fl. oz. soft cream cheese
- 2 eggs

HOW TO COOK IT

1. Heat the oven to 350 °F degrees. Lay out the parchment in 12 molds for muffins.

2. Mix together the almond flour and butter, then spread the mixture with a spoon over the forms and slightly push it inside.

3. Mix cream cheese, eggs, sweetener and vanilla extract with a mixer until smooth. Spread the spoon on top of the dough in the tins.

4. Bake in a preheated oven for 15 to 17 minutes.

5. Before you serve them, cupcakes should be refrigerated for around eight hours.

CALORIES PER SERVING:

Calories: 204. Fat: 0.74 oz. Protein: 0.17 oz. Carbs: 0.07 oz.

CHOCOLATES WITH BERRIES

How long it takes to prepare: 25 minutes
The number of serves: 12

THE INGREDIENTS:

- ♦ 4 tablespoons Solid coconut oil
- ♦ 1 cup Fresh berries mix
- ♦ 1 tablespoon Liquid coconut oil
- ♦ 2 tablespoons Cocoa powder
- ♦ 1 tablespoon Erythritol or xylitol
- ♦ 2 tablespoons Cocoa butter

HOW TO COOK IT:

1. Add solid coconut oil, cocoa butter, liquid coconut oil, salt, cocoa powder and sweetener to taste in a saucepan. Stir at low heat until finally dissolved.
2. Pour the chocolate mix into the tray and create at least 12 forms. Sprinkle berries evenly.
3. Place the tray in the fridge for about 15 minutes.
4. Store what is left in a fridge in a container with a lid.

CALORIES PER SERVING:

Calories: 61. Fat: 0.21 oz. Protein: 0.03 oz. Carbs: 0.07 oz.

KETO COOKIES WITH RASPBERRY JAM

How long it takes to prepare: 25 minutes
The number of serves: 12

THE INGREDIENTS:

- ♦ 2 cup Almond flour
- ♦ 1/4 tablespoon Xanthan gum
- ♦ 3 tablespoons of raspberry jam / sugar-free jam
- ♦ 1 Egg
- ♦ ½ tablespoon of baking powder
- ♦ 4 oz. Soft butter
- ♦ 2 oz. Erythritol or other keto-friendly sweetener
- ♦ 1 tablespoon of Vanilla extract

HOW TO COOK IT:

1. Pre-heat the oven to 370 °F degrees and place a baking sheet with parchment paper.
2. Mix flour, Xanthan gum, baking powder and salt in a small bowl. Put aside.
3. Beat the butter and sweetener together until the mass gets airy.
4. Add egg and vanilla extract.
5. Add the flour mixture and mix well.
6. Divide the dough into 12 balls. Place them on the prepared baking sheet.
7. 7. Click on the center of each ball to make a cookie. In the center of each place ½ tablespoon of jam.
8. Bake the cookies for around 10 minutes until the edges are light golden brown.
9. Allow to cool until the jam hardens.

CALORIES PER SERVING:

Calories: 168. Fat: 0.56 oz. Protein: 0.14 oz. Carbs: 0.07 oz.

CHOCOLATE BROWNIE IN A MUG

How long it takes to prepare: 25 minutes
The number of serves: 12

THE INGREDIENTS:

- ◆ 1 big egg
- ◆ 2 tablespoons of almond flour
- ◆ ½ tablespoon of baking powder
- ◆ 2 tablespoons of unsweetened cocoa powder
- ◆ 1 tablespoon of butter or coconut oil
- ◆ ½ tablespoon of Vanilla extract
- ◆ 1 tablespoon of Stevia

HOW TO COOK IT:

1. Put oil into one big cup or into two small shapes. Put it or them aside.

2. Add all ingredients to a small bowl and mix with a small whisk until smooth.

3. Pour the dough into the form. Place in the microwave for about 1 minute.

CALORIES PER SERVING:

Calories: 140. Fat: 0.32 oz. Protein: 0.39 oz. Carbs: 0.11 oz.

LEMON BLUEBERRY KETO-CAKES

How long it takes to prepare: 25 minutes
The number of serves: 12

THE INGREDIENTS:

Dough:

- 4 eggs
- 3/4 cup of fatty coconut milk
- 1 tablespoon of pure vanilla extract
- ½ cup Coconut flour
- 1½ tablespoon of Xylitol
- 1 tablespoon of baking powder
- ½ tablespoon of Xanthan gum
- 1/8 tablespoon of Pink Himalayan salt
- 3 tablespoon of herbal unsalted butter, melted
- 3/4 cup Fresh blueberries

Lemon icing:

- 1 lemon, juice and zest
- 5 tablespoons of powdered (non-granular) Stevia or xylitol

HOW TO COOK IT:

1. Pre-heat the oven to 370 °F degrees.
2. Mix eggs, coconut milk and vanilla.
3. Add coconut flour, xylitol, baking powder, Xanthan gum and salt, and beat well. Add melted butter and mix it again.
4. Add fresh blueberries carefully.
5. Fill 12 cupcakes with dough.
6. Place a baking tray with forms on the central grid of the oven. Bake them for about 20 minutes.
7. 7. Take away from the oven and cool down.

8. Mix lemon juice with powdered sweetener. Pour each cupcake with a small amount of icing. Garnish with fresh lemon peel.

CALORIES PER SERVING:

Calories: 136. Fat: 0.25 oz. Protein: 0.32 oz. Carbs: 0.21 oz.

BONUS!

YOU CAN LOSE AROUND 20 POUNDS IN 3 WEEKS:

A 3-WEEK PLAN

WEEK 1:

The first week should be very simple. It will help you to adapt to a new lifestyle. You don't need it to be a difficult change, because it will be hard to just get rid of your desires to eat the food that you are used to.

When you start the diet, you will definitely feel the first sign of it called the "keto flu": you will experience headaches, brain fogginess, and fatigue. Make sure that you get a lot of liquid. Being on the keto diet, you should be aware that you will urinate a lot. With urine, you will lose a lot of electrolytes, that's why you are sure to get constant headaches. In order to get rid of them, you should take salt and water in high enough levels because it is very important, which will allow your body to re-hydrate and supply your electrolytes again through salt and water.

And here are first general guidelines as to what you should have at various mealtimes during the day. Later a comprehensive list of day-to-day nutrition will be presented.

What to have for your breakfast:
In the morning, you will definitely want to cook something quick, easy, and tasty. You can make something in the evening, beforehand and it will last you for the entire week. The first week is about simplicity.

What to have for your lunch:
Mostly, it will be salad and meat, and that's it. You can also eat canned chicken/fish. If you do use canned meats, try to read the labels and get the one that uses the least preservatives and additives

What to have for your dinner:
Dinner will consist of a mix of greens (usually broccoli and spinach) with some kind of meat.

WEEK # 1 DETAILED PLAN TO FOLLOW:

DAY 1

Calories in total: 1,650 Kcal
Fat: 132 g / 4.65 oz
Protein: 88 g / 3.10 oz
Carb: 14 g / 0.49 oz

What to have for breakfast:
Spinach with feta cheese
A cup of coffee with two tablespoons of whipped cream

What to have for lunch:
Egg salad (2 eggs, mayo, some mustard, salt and pepper)
2 bacon slices
4 lettuce leaves

What to have for a snack:
20-24 raw almond nuts

What to have for dinner:
9 oz of grilled chicken
2 cups of chopped lettuce salad
3/4 cup casserole with cauliflower
2 tablespoons of Caesar salad (without sugar)

What to have for dessert:
Two square pieces of dark bitter chocolate - 90%

Calories in total: 1,630 Kcal
Fat: 126 g / 4.44 oz
Protein: 88 g / 3.10 oz
Carb: 18.5 g / 0.65 oz

What to have for breakfast:
Spinach with feta cheese
A cup of coffee with two tablespoons of whipped cream

What to have for lunch:
4 tablespoons of chopped lettuce salad
2 tablespoons of Caesar salad dressing (without sugar)
One small portion of chicken meat

What to have for a snack:
20-24 raw almond nuts

What to have for dinner:
1 Italian sausage, cooked and sliced
1 portion of boiled broccoli
1 piece of butter
2 tablespoons of grated Parmesan cheese

What to have for dessert:
Two square pieces of dark bitter chocolate - 90%

Calories in total: 1,512 Kcal
Fat: 119 g / 4.20 oz
Protein: 78 g / 2.75 oz
Carb: 18 g / 0.63 oz

What to have for breakfast:
Two pieces of fried bacon
Two pieces of hard cheese
A cup of coffee with two tablespoons of whipped cream

What to have for lunch:
1 Italian sausage, cooked and sliced
¾ cauliflower casserole

What to have for a snack:
One cup of bone broth

What to have for dinner:
One and a half cups of pumpkin pasta with minced meat and spices
Two portions of raw spinach

What to have for dessert:
Two square pieces of dark bitter chocolate - 90%

BONUS

Calories in total: 1,386 Kcal
Fat: 112 g / 3.95 oz
Protein: 69 g / 2.43 oz
Carb: 19.5 g / 0.68 oz

What to have for breakfast:
Spinach frittata with feta cheese
A cup of coffee with two tablespoons of whipped cream

What to have for lunch:
One and a half cups of pumpkin pasta with minced meat and spicy sauce

What to have for dinner:
1/2 bowl of antipasto salad
4 meatballs with dried tomatoes and feta cheese
2 portions of raw spinach
1 tablespoon of Italian dressing (without sugar)

What to have for dessert:
Two square pieces of dark bitter chocolate - 90%

Calories in total: 1,649 Kcal
Fat: 132 g / 4.65 oz
Protein: 81 g / 2.85 oz
Carb: 18.5 g / 0.65 oz

What to have for breakfast:
2 cheese fritters
2 pieces of fried bacon

What to have for lunch:
1/2 bowl of antipasto salad
4 meatballs with dried tomatoes and feta cheese

What to have for a snack:
Five sticks of celery with 2 tbsp. almond

What to have for dinner:
1 Keto Cuban Pot Roast
2 portions of chopped lettuce salad
2 tablespoons of sour cream
1/4 cup of crushed cheddar

What to have for dessert:
Two square pieces of dark bitter chocolate - 90%

BONUS

Calories in total: 1,604 Kcal
Fat: 122 g / 4.30 oz
Protein: 89 g / 3.14 oz
Carb: 19.5 g / 0.68 oz

What to have for breakfast:
3 eggs, fried or scrambled
One teaspoon of oil
A cup of coffee with two tablespoons of whipped cream

What to have for lunch:
1 Keto Cuban Pot Roast
2 portions of chopped lettuce salad
2 tablespoons of sour cream
1/4 cup of crushed cheddar

What to have for a snack:
One cup of bone broth

What to have for dinner:
1/2 cups of pumpkin pasta with minced meat and spicy sauce
2 portions of raw spinach
1 tablespoon of ranch sauce (without sugar)

What to have for dessert:
Nothing!

DAY 7

Calories in total: 1,609 Kcal
Fat: 128 g / 4.51 oz
Protein: 90 g / 3.17 oz
Carb: 18 g / 0.63 oz

What to have for breakfast:

2 cheese fritters
2 pieces of bacon
A cup of coffee with two tablespoons of whipped cream

What to have for lunch:

1 Keto Cuban Pot Roast
2 portions of chopped lettuce salad
2 tablespoons of sour cream
1/4 cup of crushed cheddar

What to have for a snack:

One cup of bone broth

What to have for dinner:

1 Keto Cuban Pot Roast
2 portions of chopped lettuce salad
2 tablespoons of sour cream
1/4 cup of grated cheddar cheese

What to have for dessert:

Two square pieces of dark bitter chocolate - 90%

BONUS

WEEK # 2

Now we come to the second week of our diet.

DAY 1 WEEK 2

Calories in total: 1,622 Kcal
Fat: 128 g / 4.51 oz
Protein: 72 g / 2.54 oz
Carb: 16.5 g / 0.58 oz

What to have for breakfast:
2 Cream Cheese Pancakes
2 pieces of cooked bacon
a cup of hot coffee adding two tablespoons of cream

What to have for lunch:
1 cup of Jalapeno Popper Soup
1 Jalapeno & Cheddar Muffin

What to have for a snack:
One cup of bone broth

What to have for dinner:
1/4 Flax Pizza
2 cups raw baby spinach
1 tablespoon of ranch dressing (sugar-free)

What to have for dessert:
Two square pieces of dark bitter chocolate - 90%

Calories in total: 1,657 Kcal
Fat: 122 g / 4.30 oz
Protein: 89 g / 3.14 oz
Carb: 16.5 g / 0.58 oz

What to have for breakfast:
2 eggs (you can choose either scrambled or fried ones)
1 tablespoon of butter
2 pieces of cooked bacon
a cup of hot coffee adding two tablespoons of cream

What to have for lunch:
1/4 Flax Pizza

What to have for a snack:
1/2 avocado with salt and pepper

What to have for dinner:
1 Paprika Chicken Thigh with sauce
1/2 portion of Cheesy Cauliflower Puree
2 portions of raw spinach
1 tablespoon of ranch dressing (sugar-free)

What to have for dessert:
Two square pieces of dark bitter chocolate - 90%

Calories in total: 1,839 Kcal
Fat: 154 g / 5.43 oz
Protein: 86 g / 3.03 oz
Carb: 17.5 g / 0.62 oz

What to have for breakfast:
2 Cream Cheese Pancakes
2 pieces of cooked bacon
a cup of hot coffee adding two tablespoons of cream

What to have for lunch:
1 Paprika Chicken Thigh with sauce
1/2 portion of Cheesy Cauliflower Puree

What to have for a snack:
1/2 avocado with salt and pepper

What to have for dinner:
1 cup of Jalapeno Popper Soup
2 tablespoons of Italian dressing (sugar-free)
1 Jalapeno & Cheddar Muffin
2 cups of chopped lettuce

What to have for dessert:
Two square pieces of dark bitter chocolate - 90%

Calories in total: 1,843 Kcal
Fat: 141 g / 4.97 oz
Protein: 82 g / 2.90 oz
Carb: 18 g / 0.63 oz

What to have for breakfast:
1 Jalapeno & Cheddar Muffin
2 eggs (scrambled or fried)
1 tablespoon of butter
2 pieces of cooked bacon
a cup of hot coffee adding two tablespoons of cream

What to have for lunch:
1/4 Flax Pizza

What to have for a snack:
1/2 avocado with salt and pepper

What to have for dinner:
1 cup of Jalapeno Popper Soup
1 Jalapeno & Cheddar Muffin
2 portions of chopped lettuce
2 tablespoons of ranch dressing (sugar-free)

What to have for dessert:
Two square pieces of dark bitter chocolate - 90%

BONUS

Calories in total: 1,618 Kcal
Fat: 106 g / 3.74 oz
Protein: 89 g / 3.14 oz
Carb: 18 g / 0.63 oz

What to have for breakfast:
2 Cream Cheese Pancakes
2 pieces of cooked bacon
a cup of hot coffee adding two tablespoons of cream

What to have for lunch:
1/4 Flax Pizza
Plus:
2 cups of raw baby spinach
1 tablespoon of Italian dressing (sugar-free)

What to have for a snack:
1 cup of bone broth

What to have for dinner:
3 Meatballs alla Parmigiana
2 cups of chopped romaine lettuce
2 tablespoon of Italian dressing (sugar free)

What to have for dessert:
Two square pieces of dark bitter chocolate - 90%

BONUS

Calories in total: 1,892 Kcal
Fat: 153 g / 5.40 oz
Protein: 100 g / 3.53 oz
Carb: 16 g / 0.56 oz

What to have for breakfast:
1 Jalapeno & Cheddar Muffin
2 eggs (scrambled or fried)
1 tablespoon of butter
2 pieces of cooked bacon
a cup of hot coffee adding two tablespoons of cream

What to have for lunch:
1 cup of Jalapeno Popper Soup
1 Jalapeno & Cheddar Muffin

What to have for a snack:
1 cup of bone broth

What to have for dinner:
1 Paprika Chicken Thigh with sauce
1/2 portion of Cheesy Cauliflower Puree
2 cups of chopped lettuce
2 tablespoons of Italian dressing (sugar-free)

What to have for dessert:
Two square pieces of dark bitter chocolate - 90%

BONUS

Calories in total: 1,724 Kcal
Fat: 118 g / 4.16 oz
Protein: 95 g / 3.35 oz
Carb: 19 g / 0.67 oz

What to have for breakfast:
2 Cream Cheese Pancakes
2 pieces of cooked bacon
a cup of hot coffee adding two tablespoons of cream

What to have for lunch:
3 Meatballs alla Parmigiana
2 cups of chopped romaine lettuce

What to have for a snack:
1 cup of bone broth

What to have for dinner:
1 Paprika Chicken Thigh with sauce
1/2 portion of Cheesy Cauliflower Puree
2 cups of chopped lettuce
2 tablespoons of Italian dressing (sugar-free)

What to have for dessert:
Nothing!

BONUS

WEEK # 3

And now we come to the third final week. By now you will have noticed that you are feeling better and the results have become visible. Enjoy your third week of healthy living with the keto diet!

DAY 1

Calories in total:
1,775 calories
5.22 oz/ 148 g fat
0.65 oz/ 18.5g net carb
3.07 oz / 87 g protein)

What to have for breakfast:
2 Cream Cheese Pancakes
2 pieces of cooked bacon
a cup of hot coffee adding two tablespoons of cream

What to have for a snack:
12 raw almonds

What to have for lunch:
2 Cream Cheese Pancakes
4 slices of ham
2 slices of deli cheddar cheese
1 tablespoon of mayo:
Instructions:
Spread the mayonnaise onto the pancakes, and then put 2 slices of ham and 1 slice of cheese on each of the pancakes. Add spinach if you like.

What to have for a snack:
1 piece of cheese

What to have for dinner:
3/4 cup Cheesy Chipotle Cauliflower
2 Green Enchilada Meatballs

What to have for dessert:
1 Raspberry Cheesecake Bar

Calories in total:
1,410 calories,
3.99 oz/ 113 g fat
0.67 oz/ 19 g net carb,
3.00 oz/ 85g protein

What to have for breakfast:
1 serving of Ham and Cheese Frittata
a cup of hot coffee adding two tablespoons of cream

What to have for a snack:
1/2 avocado with salt and pepper

What to have for lunch:
4 Green Enchilada Meatballs

What to have for a snack:
2 slices of cheese

What to have for dinner:
1 and 3/4 cup Sausage, Kale & Squash Soup
1 Jalapeno & Cheddar Muffin

What to have for dessert:
1 Raspberry Cheesecake Bar

Calories in total:
1,619 calories,
4.69 oz/ 133g fat,
0.58 oz/ 16.5g net carbs,
2.32 oz/ 66g protein

What to have for breakfast:
2 Cream Cheese Pancakes
2 pieces of cooked bacon
a cup of hot coffee adding two tablespoons of cream

What to have for a snack:
1/2 avocado with salt and pepper

What to have for lunch:
1 serving of Ham and Cheese Frittata
2 portions of chopped romaine lettuce
2 tablespoons of Italian dressing (sugar-free)

What to have for a snack:
12 raw almonds

What to have for dinner:
3/4 cup of Cheesy Chipotle Cauliflower
2 Green Enchilada Meatballs

What to have for dessert:
1 Raspberry Cheesecake Bar

BONUS

Calories in total:
1,279 calories
3.35 oz/ 95g fat
0.67 oz/ 19g net carbs
2.05 oz/ 58g protein

What to have for breakfast:
1 serving of Ham and Cheese Frittata
2 pieces of cooked bacon
a cup of hot coffee adding two tablespoons of cream

What to have for a snack:
12 raw almonds

What to have for lunch:
1 3/4 cup of Sausage, Kale & Squash Soup

What to have for a snack:
1/2 avocado with salt and pepper

What to have for dinner:
1 serving of Chicken Stir Fry
2 cups of chopped romaine lettuce
2 tablespoon of Italian dressing (sugar-free)

What to have for dessert:
1 Raspberry Cheesecake Bar

DAY 5

Calories in total:
1,669 calories
4.59 oz/ 130g fat
0.71 oz/ 20g net carbs
2.86 oz/ 81g protein

What to have for breakfast:
2 Cream Cheese Pancakes
2 pieces of cooked bacon
a cup of hot coffee adding two tablespoons of cream

What to have for a snack:
1/2 avocado with salt and pepper

What to have for lunch:
1 serving of Chicken Stir Fry

What to have for a snack:
1 serving of Ham and Cheese Frittata

What to have for dinner:
3/4 cup Cheesy Chipotle Cauliflower
2 Green Enchilada Meatballs

What to have for dessert:
1 Raspberry Cheesecake Bar

Calories in total:
1,447 calories
4.02 oz/ 114g fat
0.63 oz/ 18g net carbs
3.03 oz/ 86g protein

What to have for breakfast:
1 serving of Ham and Cheese Frittata
2 pieces of cooked bacon
a cup of hot coffee adding two tablespoons of cream

What to have for a snack:
12 raw almonds

What to have for lunch:
4 Green Enchilada Meatballs

What to have for a snack:
2 slices of cheese

What to have for dinner:
1 3/4 cup Sausage, Kale & Squash Soup
2 cups of chopped romaine lettuce
2 tablespoon of Italian dressing (sugar-free)

What to have for dessert:
1 Raspberry Cheesecake Bar

BONUS

DAY 7

Calories in total:
1,712 calories
4.88 oz/ 138g fat
0.69 oz/ 19.5g net carbs
3.25 oz/ 92g protein

What to have for breakfast:
2 Cream Cheese Pancakes
2 pieces of cooked bacon
a cup of hot coffee adding two tablespoons of cream

What to have for a snack:
1 slice of cheese

What to have for lunch:
4 Green Enchilada Meatballs

What to have for a snack:
2 slices of cheese

What to have for dinner:
1 3/4 cup Sausage, Kale & Squash Soup
2 cups of chopped romaine lettuce
2 tablespoon of Italian dressing (sugar-free)

What to have for dessert:
1 Raspberry Cheesecake Bar

BONUS

CONCLUSION

CONCLUSION

At the beginning you might think it is very difficult to follow the Keto Diet. However, the popularity of healthy and green food is becoming wider, which makes it simpler to find high-quality low-carb products.

You should follow the plan of the diet. The best results can be achieved by those who strictly limit the intake of carbohydrates. Get rid of extra sugar and sweeteners in your diet.

Drink a lot of water and replenish electrolytes. Most of the common problems are caused by dehydration and lack of electrolytes. When you start the keto diet, make sure you drink enough water, add some fresh juice to your diet. If you still have some side effects, so you should get electrolytes as a separate supplement.

Keep a nutrition diary of yours. Going beyond the acceptable carbo-level is very easy. Hidden carbohydrates are found in almost every product you consume. Recording what you eat helps to check the amount of net carbohydrates consumed and you will feel responsible for your diet.

The keto diet is a low-carb, high-fat diet.

It will decrease your blood sugar and insulin levels, shift metabolism from carbohydrates to fats and ketones. **Be healthy and keep fit!**

DISCLAIMER

This book contains opinions and ideas of the author and is meant to teach the reader informative and helpful knowledge while due care should be taken by the user in the application of the information provided. The instructions and strategies are possibly not right for every reader and there is no guarantee that they work for everyone. Using this book and implementing the information/recipes therein contained is explicitly your own responsibility and risk. This work with all its contents, does not guarantee correctness, completion, quality or correctness of the provided information. Misinformation or misprints cannot be completely eliminated.

Design: Oliviaprodesign

Picture: Kiian Oksana / www.shutterstock.com